The How Healing Happens Series

Energetic Pampering

Quantum Face-Lift

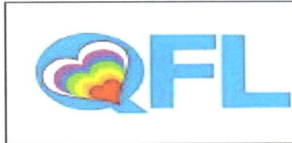

For the Fun of It

Trudy Baker QHP, QHI

Quantum Face-Lift: A series of self-healing techniques and exercises that foster beautiful facial appearance

ISBN: 978-0-9916848-5-4

DEDICATION

To women of all ages, but especially to those of us,
Boomers, who are always fighting wrinkles and crepey skin.

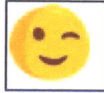

ACKNOWLEDGMENTS

The methods used are a combination of ancient and modern healing modalities. The hand positions are similar to those used in an Access Consciousness' Facelift and a Pranic Facelift. Thanks to Laurence Moore and Zaid Bhabha for assistance in fine tuning the techniques. Thanks to Miriam Orta, her daughters Lee-ann and Kathleen and the ladies in Laredo and San Antonio, Texas for being part of the first run of the Quantum Face-Lift workshop. Their participation and input have been extremely valuable. Special thanks to Miriam for allowing the use of her picture on the cover and throughout the book. A special thumbs up for S.V. Bella and her colleagues for their input as cosmetologists. Thanks to Sam Adams for giving me the extra encouragement to run with the Quantum-Face-Lift Project, for his marketing and web design expertise. Photography credits to Sandoval El Bello Arte, by Nancy & Roberto Sandoval. Cover design by Panagiotis Lampridis.

Above all, I am much appreciative of my husband Everett's editorial input, support and patience with me for all the time it kept me at my desk

PRAISE FOR QUANTUM FACE-LIFTS

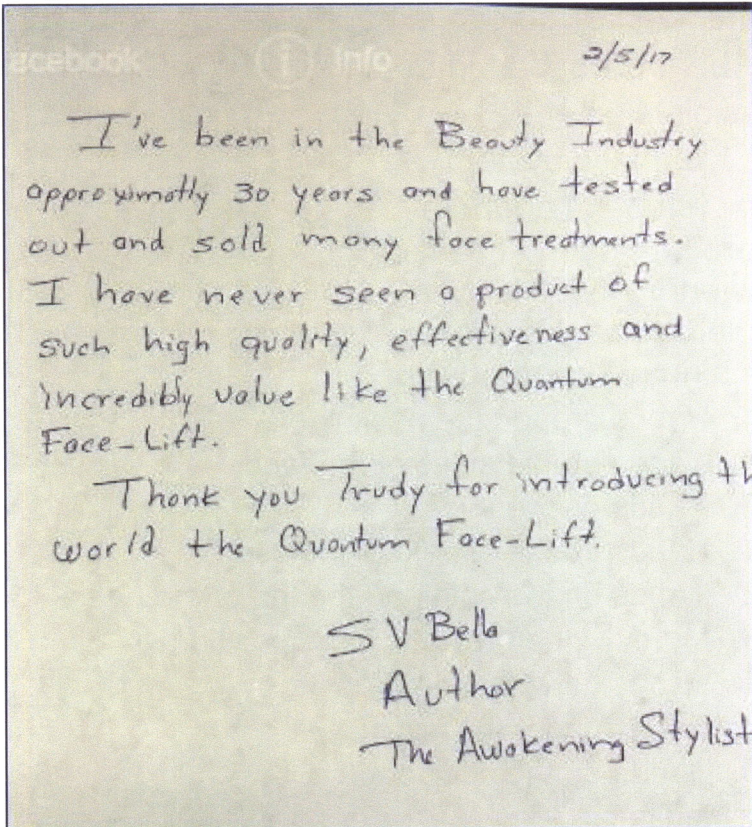

2/5/17

I've been in the Beauty Industry approximatly 30 years and have tested out and sold many face treatments. I have never seen a product of such high quality, effectiveness and incredibly value like the Quantum Face-Lift.

Thank you Trudy for introducing th world the Quantum Face-Lift.

S V Bella
Author
The Awakening Stylist

TABLE OF CONTENTS

INTRODUCTION

The material covered was first introduced as a weekend workshop under the title Quantum Face-Lift to a group of cosmetologists who were interested in a value-added item to offer their clientele. They showed me the importance of making people feel good as well as look good. People who feel good show an inner confidence that increases their power to look good. People who are pleased with their appearance when looking in the mirror immediately feel better about themselves. I also learned the difference between a facelift and a facial. The Oxford dictionary defines a facial as a beauty treatment for the face, often including the application of make-up. Special offers for a facial may also include a manicure. A facelift is defined as a cosmetic surgical operation to remove unwanted wrinkles by tightening the skin of the face to create a youthful appearance. Non-surgical facelifts are done with the use of chemicals such as Botox injected into the skin or into the muscles. The result is a tightening of the skin by collagen stimulation and skin firming.

A Quantum Face-Lift is an effective process that smoothens, tightens and rejuvenates the skin on your face without the use of make-up, chemical injections or surgery. People who have taken the workshop report increased energy, stability, and clarity. Unexpected, but marvelous side effects!   Imagine, to achieve such results without surgery, without injections, without drugs!

Reading the booklet will introduce you to all the techniques, hand positions and energy work needed to do a Quantum Face-Lift for yourself. Cosmetologists will be able to integrate the procedures into their treatments for their clients.

Reading the booklet may well encourage you to plan to attend a workshop and take the opportunity to do a complete Quantum Face-Lift as well as receive a complete personal session yourself. Enjoy a Participatory workshop! The Quantum Facelift works effectively and professionally in spas, massage practices, anti-aging and wellness centers worldwide. The skills learned are a fabulous addition to any beauty therapist business and massage therapist wishing to extend services to their clientele.

A Quantum Face-Lift is a wonderful way to rejuvenate the face and reverse the appearance of aging. What if you could have a natural facelift instead of surgical procedures or the use of chemicals such as Botox?

Who wouldn't like to have bragging rights about

– a lessening of lines and wrinkles

– improved eyesight

– firmness and toning of facial muscles and overall skin

– healing and reversal of the scarring process

– healthier skin and overall appearance

Learning to use a Quantum Facelift has the potential for an upgrade in your life and in your practice as a beautician exceeding any expectations you ever dreamed of.

SOME RESULTS YOU CAN EXPECT

I taught the Quantum Face-Lift techniques to a group of cosmetologists in Laredo, Texas, in July 2016. The pictures below show the effect the weekend had on my face and neck.

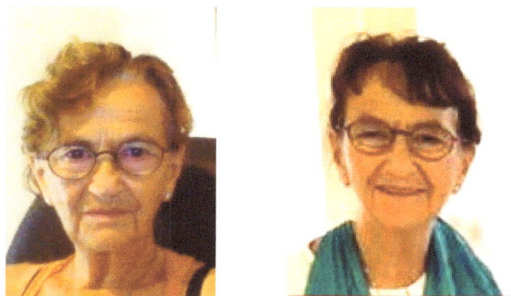

The picture on the left was taken while I was putting together the presentation, the month before going to Laredo. The second picture at the graduation ceremony at the end of the workshop. I used no make-up, no product of any kind. No Photoshop effects were added to either picture. It's all energy work. The results you see were after only one weekend. It was an intensive weekend: 4 hours Friday night, 12 hours on Saturday, from 9:00 am till 10:00 pm, with a few short breaks, and again from 10:00 am till

5:00 pm on Sunday. There were 14 of us participating in the workshop. The vibrations singly and together really revved up during the time of the workshop. All the participants were pleased with the end results on their faces.

THE BENEFITS OF A QUANTUM FACE-LIFT

The benefits of a Quantum Face-Lift (QFL) are manifold. People have experienced unexpected results almost immediately, and sometimes weeks later more benefits become evident. It's not the same for everyone. Much depends on one's expectations and focus as well as on the commitment to continue using the program. It is not a one-time fix, rather a commitment to self-care on a whole new level. It's comparable to a fitness program. We all know that one trip to the gym is not going to remove those unwanted inches from our waste-line, nor tone our legs and firm up our flabby underarms. Or think of a nutrition plan you've been advised to follow to improve your life. Reading a cookbook with many nourishing vegan recipes is not going to do the trick. Any such program takes effort and prolonged practice before you see any results. The Quantum Face-Lift techniques and methods work best with repeated practice.The program is really very pleasant. No sweat, no sore muscles, no outlay of a lot of money. Invest

20 minutes a day, just for yourself. The returns are phenomenal.

The techniques are non-invasive and the results are soft and subtle. Facial wrinkles will lessen. The skin will increase in firmness and the muscles of the face will become more toned. It gives you an overall healthier appearance. Quantum Face-lifts will decrease the tendency towards sagging jowls. It will tighten the skin on the neck. It will reduce double chins and lift drooping eyelids. Old scars may lessen, heal and reverse to new healthy looking skin. The healing process of blemishes will be stimulated, and blemishes will heal scar-free. During repeated sessions, the soft tissue on the face will improve. So will blood circulation. People with acute and chronic pain in and around the ears may experience a great sense of relief. One's eyesight will likely improve over time. All this is a result of the promotion of anti-inflammatory and anti-edematous effects that happen during a period of repeated energetic work on the face. On an energetic level, the physical function of the lymphatic system is restored. If that is not enough, remember, an energetic facial treatment simply feels good!

There is more! Some of the noted benefits of a Quantum Face-Lift are not commonly associated with a beauty treatment known as a facelift. Here's what else you may expect.

A Quantum Face-Lift may remove hormonal imbalances which cause facial acné. It will improve metabolism which will eliminate edema and puffiness. Local blood and lymph circulation will increase improving facial color. Every Quantum Face-Lift session will help reduce stress, menopause discomfort, and PMS and improve overall health and wellbeing. TMJ, trigeminal neuralgia and Bell's Palsy may be reduced. Sinus congestion and headaches will lessen. Eyes, ears, thyroid and the brain will be helped to function normally. For people of advanced age, the sessions will retard hair loss and graying.

POSSIBLE SIDE EFFECTS

Here's the small print. For most people, a Quantum Face-Lift alleviates tiredness and stress. It reduces depression. Many women who use the methods and techniques on themselves become more alert and experience a greater ability to concentrate. Tension, migraine, and stress related headaches decrease. Due to the increase in blood flow a person will likely become more active. The process alleviates earaches, jaw ache, tinnitus and sinusitis congestion. One can expect improved functionality of the lymphatic system. Bottom line: none of the side effects are negative, rather you can expect unexpected positive outcomes.

A Graduate's Note to me, a Year Later

I love to include a mini Quantum Face-Lift technique every morning in my daily facial routine. I can see it and I can feel it. I also use it with my clients at the Spa. My clients are happier than ever. A Little LOVE to pamper my clients and myself every morning makes my day. I do a full Quantum Face-Lift therapy at least once a week, and I call it "QFL, the Energetic Fountain of Youth"

Miriam Orta
Beauty Salon and Spa Owner

THE LYMPHATIC SYSTEM

The lymphatic system, also known as the immune system, is a network of tissues and organs made up of lymph vessels, lymph nodes, lymph, spleen, bone marrow and the thymus gland. It clears away infection and keeps your body fluids in balance.

How does a Quantum Face-Lift get credit for doing all the benefits mentioned above?

We engage the Life Force Energy to boost and in some cases reactivate the lymphatic system. When we "run energy" the energy follows our thoughts. Therefore, while doing a Quantum Face-Lift, think about your client's and your own Lymphatic System working at optimal capacity.

Inside our body, there is an amazing protection mechanism called the immune system or lymphatic system. It is designed to defend us against millions of bacteria, microbes, viruses, toxins and parasites that would love to invade our body. The lymphatic system is responsible for getting toxins out of the body. Running energy on the lymph

19

nodes helps the Lymphatic System to function better. Your skin benefits as toxins are being removed.

Dr. Bruno Chikly, M.D. and Doctor of Osteopathy (D.O.) writes in an article entitled "Best Face Forward: The Mini Face Lift Effects of Lymph Drainage Therapy" (Massage Magazine, February 2012), not only does lymph drainage help edema (fluid retention), it also helps with the reduction of appearance of scars and wrinkles.

By learning the position of lymph nodes on the face, neck, and chest you will know better where to place your hands.

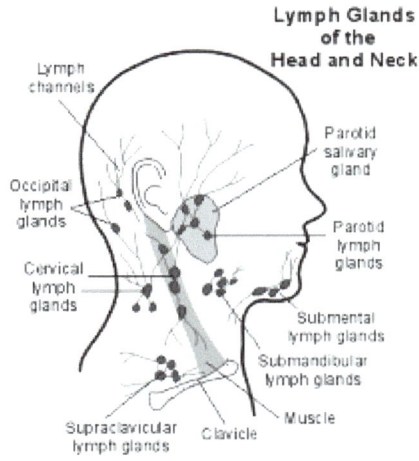

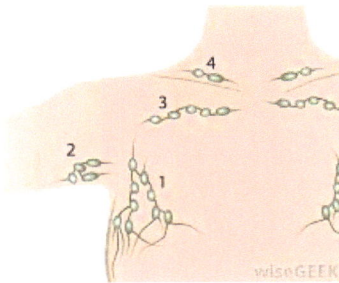

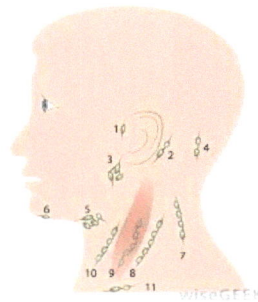

Lymph Glands
of the
Head and Neck

Lymph channels

Parotid salivary gland

Occipital lymph glands

Parotid lymph glands

Cervical lymph glands

Submental lymph glands

Submandibular lymph glands

Muscle

Supraclavicular lymph glands

Clavicle

Superficial (Surface) Lymphatics

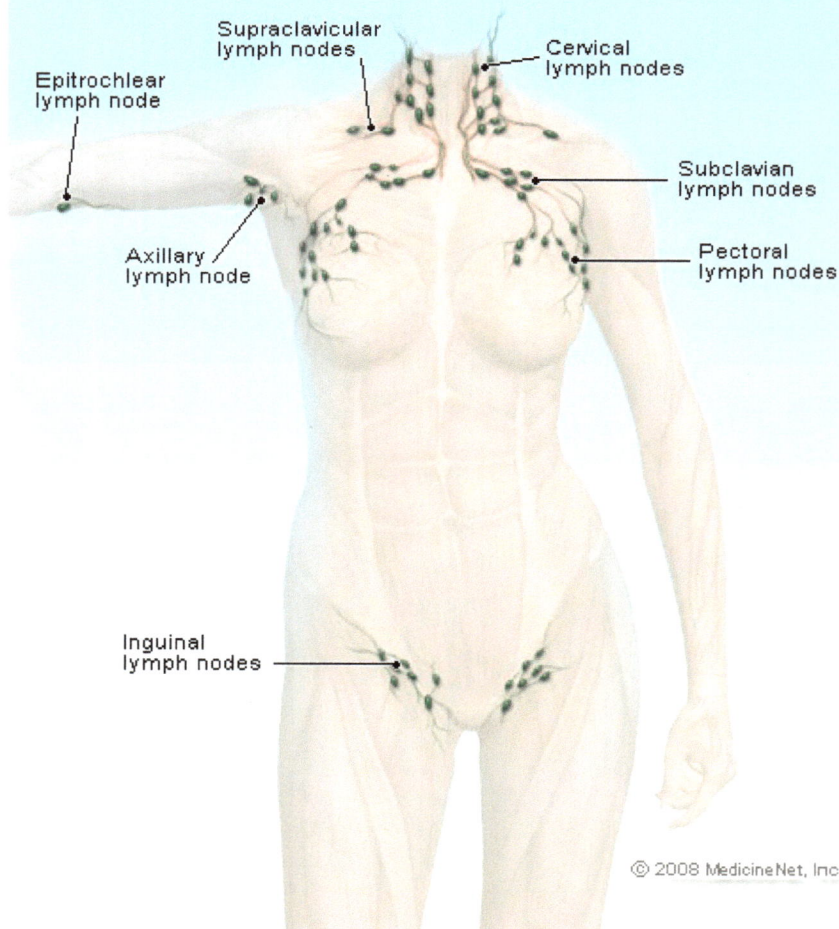

Supraclavicular
lymph nodes

Cervical
lymph nodes

Epitrochlear
lymph node

Subclavian
lymph nodes

Axillary
lymph node

Pectoral
lymph nodes

Inguinal
lymph nodes

© 2008 MedicineNet, Inc.

Lymph drainage has an anti-aging effect because it works on the parasympathetic nervous system. It promotes a deep state of relaxation to the face and body. Releasing skin tension helps to regenerate and oxygenate, thereby improving overall facial beauty. Reducing stress on the body and face also helps to relax the face, beautifying your facial appearance. The Quantum Face-Lift explained in this booklet differs from both the Pranic facial and the Access Consciousness facelift, neither of which focus on engaging the lymphatic system.

To understand the power of the immune system, all we have to do is observe what happens to anything once it dies. When something dies, its immune system (along with everything else) shuts down. In a matter of hours, a body is invaded by all sorts of bacteria, microbes, and parasites. A healthy working immune system keeps our bodies in maximum health.

WHAT HAPPENS DURING A QUANTUM FACE-LIFT SESSION

We think of it as **energetic pampering**, but it is much more than that.

Beauticians or massage therapists can add energy work to a conventional facelift. The client entrains to the practitioners' higher vibrations. Working on yourself, one entrains to one's own highest vibrations. Both you and your client drop into a state of gentle hypnosis. When working with a client the practitioners lower their voice and speak slowly to the subconscious using positive affirmations. For yourself, you mentally say positive affirmations. You and your client become receptive to the healing energies at a subconscious level. The lymphatic system begins to function better. Toxins are removed. The skin cells are being toned, regaining elasticity, and collagen levels are restored. The warmth or heat of the energy on the underlying layers of the skin breaks down worn-out collagen and stimulates the growth of new elastic cells and the production of amino acids for healthy proteins. People need 20 different amino acids to remain healthy. 12 of them are produced by our bodies, the rest are absorbed from the diet. Some sources state these essential amino acids come from meat, fish, dairy, fish, and eggs. Protein sources, such as fruits, vegetables, grains, nuts and seeds, lack one or more essential amino acids. According to this trend in research, vegans need to add supplements to their diets. Energy work strengthens your body to produce amino acids more effectively and allows the body to do a better job absorbing amino acids from the food we eat and the supplements we take.

HOW ENERGY WORK WORKS

Readers who are familiar with energy work in one or more of the following modalities such as Reiki, Quantum Touch, Pranic Healing or similar ones may want to skip this section and move on to the next.

Energy healing was a part of my life since my childhood. It came to me as natural as walking or talking. My mother and my aunt, as well as some others in the family to a greater or lesser extent, "helped people" to get well. I watched and I learned. I "helped" a pet dog get better when he was hurting. Later I "helped" my sister to clear a rather nasty eye infection by placing my hand on it and pulling out the inflammation. It worked. I was an ordinary kid, I am an ordinary person. I believe if I can do it, so can others. When I met my husband, years ago, we did not talk about energy healing. It was not on top of my agenda at that time. He did not ask about it, simply because he was not familiar with it. Over the years he observed what I did, had many questions, and now we both practice several modalities. Together we do it better than alone.

Our approach to energy work is intermodal. Although we are trained in many different modalities, we do not favor any one over another. We have experienced the ease and seamlessness with which several healing modalities integrate with each other, and wish to promote self-healing.

A basic understanding of energy work is a prerequisite for learning to do a Quantum Face-Lift. I will give a brief overview of a few techniques that may be used to acquaint yourself with sufficient background to follow the procedures and to learn to do them for yourself and others.

The first and perhaps simplest way is using meditation techniques and intention. Find a quiet spot where you will not be interrupted for a half-hour or more. Sit comfortably. A lotus position is not required, especially not for people who do not have the physical ability to sit this way for an extended period of time. Breathe a little more slowly than normal and find your quiet place inside. Pay attention to the rhythm of your breathing and follow the up and down motions the breath creates on your abdomen. Pay attention to feeling the breath going in and out over your lower lip. If external thoughts come in, acknowledge them and let them go. Say to yourself: "OK, I'm thinking about that now. It can wait till later," and focus your attention on your breathing again. Once you begin to feel more relaxed find your place of highest focus. Internally say to yourself, "It is my intention to be in touch with the Life Force Energy." Pay attention to how your body feels. You may feel a warming sensation all over. You may feel a slight tickling sensation. You may feel nothing at all. With some practice, you will learn to go through these steps in less than a minute, and you will very likely begin to have a sense of connectedness with all that is.

Some people may like to try what is called the 'sweep and breathe' method of Quantum Touch. Stand with your feet about shoulder-width apart and the knees slightly bent and relaxed. Pretend someone is gently caressing your skin, starting at the feet and slowly moving upward to the top of your head. From there, move down across the shoulders, along your arms, and out your fingertips. Coordinate your breathing and the caressing motion. Breathe in when the caressing goes up. Breathe out when going down. With some practice this can all be done in your imagination, creating an energetic warmth or prickling all over your body. Just keep breathing and enjoy the feeling.

Personally, I like using my variation of a Shamanic Earth – Star meditation. Stand relaxed. Raise your arms with palms facing upward. Focus your thoughts on a favorite star, on the heavens or the Divine. Invite the energies of the sky to enter into your being, through the palms of your hands, through the crown of your head and through every pore of your skin. Allow the sensations to flow through your body. Now bring your arms down with palms facing towards the earth. Focus your thoughts down into the center of the earth and invite the energy of the earth to enter into your being, through the palms of your hands, through the soles of your feet and through every pore of your skin. Invite the energies of the skies and the energies of the earth to blend into your heart space and amplify them with the love of your heart. Pay attention to how your body feels.

Each of the above techniques may be done with your eyes closed or open. When you are completely relaxed, simply draw your attention back to your surroundings and take in the physical sights and sounds around you. You are back in the here and now. Neither of the methods is necessarily better or easier than the other. I invite you to try all three, play around with them and you will know what works best for you. Experiment. Wonder. Enjoy.

Each time before doing a Quantum Face-Lift tune into the Life Force Energy field using one of the methods above, or your own preferred way.

GUIDELINES

Remove all make-up before starting a Quantum Face-Lift session. Also take off all earrings and other facial jewelry, necklaces, rings and bracelets. You can work over or under clothing, depending on the type of clothing, yet wearing a simple T-shirt may be most convenient. All positions are hands-on, without any pressure. Use a very light touch or near-touch. We teach 9 hand positions. No particular order is preferable over another. It is advisable to start with the area of your face where you personally would most like to see changes happen. You can initially follow the order of the positions as they are presented here, and once you are familiar with all positions, work out a routine best suitable for yourself.

If you are a beautician or a massage therapist working with clients ask the client what part of the face they are most concerned about and start there. Always tell your client when you are ready to move to another area of the face. Starting with the clients' preference makes for an easy energy flow. It is also a good idea to keep continuous contact with the client, leaving one hand in the current position while moving your other hand to a new position. It makes for a smooth continuous session. The more familiar you become with the work, the more you can personalize your session, following your intuition. It is a good idea to keep up a conversation with the client. Speak just a bit more slowly than usually in low tones. Ask for feedback. Does the client feel the energy? Keep her involved.

THE NINE (9) HAND POSITIONS

Before starting a Quantum Face-Lift session take a few moments to go to your quiet space and 'turn on' the energy. Use either one of the three methods explained above or your own favorite method, to connect with the Life Force Energy: a. meditation combined with intention, b. Quantum Touch' sweep and breathe technique or c. the Shamanic earth star meditation. Allow the energy to flow through your body. Imagine it. Feel it. And make it real.

1. Hands around the neck

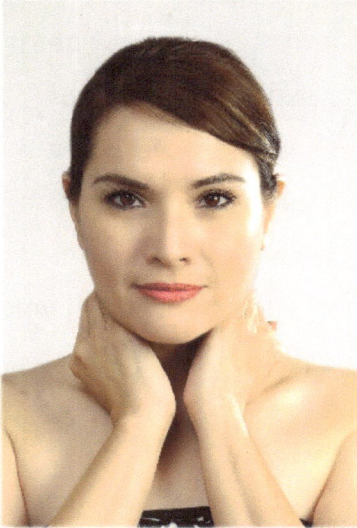

Figure 1 working on self

Place your hands to cover as much of the neck as possible, including under the chin. Your fingertips should not touch. Allow the energy to flow through your body. Imagine it. Feel it. And make it real. Hold the position and run energy for 5 minutes. Running energy under the chin impacts the lymphatic system. The position will reduce swollen glands. Do some multi- tasking: a. feel the energy, b. focus on the lymphatic system functioning at full capacity and c. set your

34

intention to have beautiful skin, healthy skin, and smooth skin. Allow the energy to flow through your body. Imagine it. Feel it. And make it real. You may notice the flow of the energy throughout your whole body.

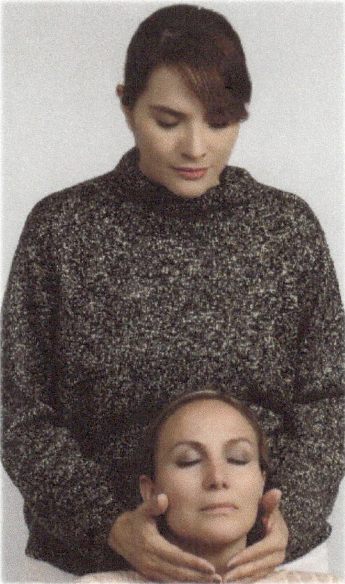

Figure 2 working on client

When you are working with a client, look for any presence of any swollen glands on the neck of the client. Carefully alert her attention to what you see. After the session, ask your client to have another look in the mirror. The instant

35

result will give her and all her friends' confidence in the process.

Positive outcomes

There is a positive carry-over effect for all neck issues. The SternoCleidoMastoid (SCM) is the large muscle in the neck. It hardly ever hurts itself, yet is responsible for many issues. They include a migraine, sinus headache, atypical facial neuralgia, trigeminal neuralgia, arthritis of the sternoclavicular joint, ataxia, multiple sclerosis (MS), brain lesions, tumors, and other similar conditions. A welcome side-effect of doing a Quantum Face-Lift will be a reduction and easing of any of the above-mentioned issues. The thyroid gland, situated in the neck will also benefit. Running energy on the thyroid will positively affect either an over-active or an under-active thyroid. As a result, you may experience a stabilization of any weight control issues.

2. Hands on the sides of the face

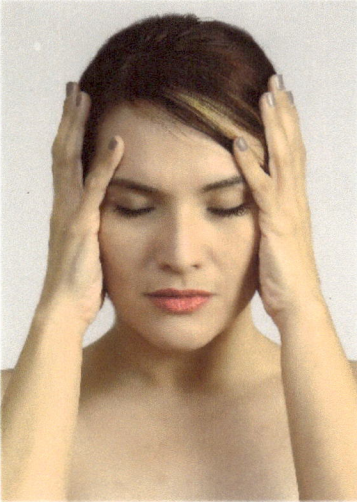

Figure 3 working on self

Place your fingers alongside the edge of the eyes on both sides of the face. Your palms cover the edges of the sphenoid bone, the temples, and the jaw. Allow the energy to flow through your body. Imagine it. Feel it. And make it real. Hold the position and run energy for 5 minutes. This position obviously intends to smoothen the skin and have the crow's feet disappear from the outer edge of the eyes. It will, and it does much more.

37

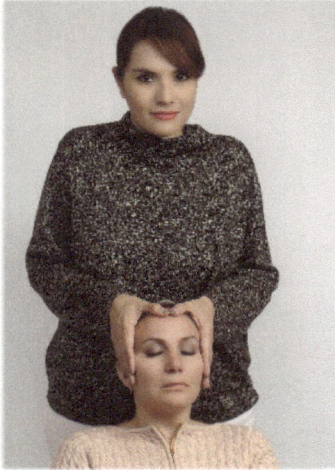

Figure 4 working on client

Positive outcomes

Running energy while your hands are on the side of your face may reduce tinnitus and remove TMJ discomfort. The position also adjusts the pelvic balance on account of the fact that the energy you are running will have a positive effect on the sphenoid bone. In chiropractic jargon, the sphenoid bone has been called the GOD bone, "**G**eometry **O**f **D**ivinity". The Sphenoid is a butterfly or bat-like shaped bone behind the eyes. It has a section, the Vomer, that rests along the upper side of the hard palette and articulates with the Occipital bone at the base of the skull. It, in turn, articulates with the spine which connects to the hip bones, which, if unbalanced, will adjust to their proper position.

The sphenoid bone flexes with each inhalation and exhalation. The hydraulic action of the cerebral spinal fluid causes the sphenoid to rock or flex toward the feet and back. In some cases where it is stuck or erratic, it will now become free. As the sphenoid begins to relax pressure on the pituitary may also be released. The significance is that the rocking motion of the sphenoid pumps the pituitary gland, which is the primary, and controlling gland in the body. A properly rocking sphenoid can have a direct bearing on the endocrine system's function. The proper functioning of the pituitary gland may dramatically improve your overall health.

3. Hands on the eyes

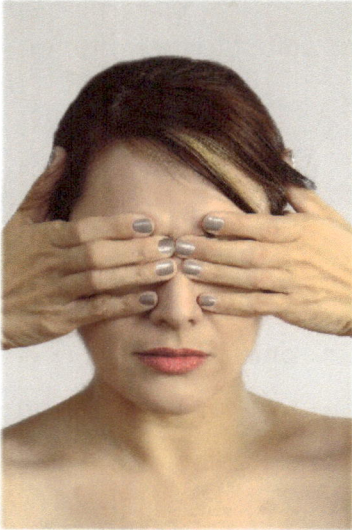

Figure 5 working on self

Place your fingers over your eyes with your thumbs pointing up. Allow the energy to flow through your body. Imagine it. Feel it. And make it real. Hold the position and run energy for 5 minutes. It may be a difficult position to hold on one's own face. Alternatively, do it while lying down on a bed or a wide massage table so you can rest your elbows on a couple of pillows placed beside your head and shoulders. The outcome is the removal of wrinkles and crow's feet

40

around the eyes. It reduces puffiness under the eyes. It removes dark circles (bags) under the eyes.

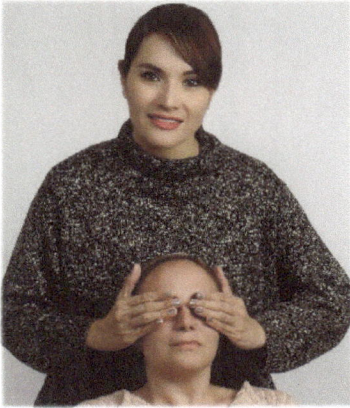

Figure 6 working on client

Depending on the relative size of the practitioner's hands and the client's face, the palms may cover most of the face.

Positive outcomes

The positive side effects may include improved eyesight, improved night vision, and reduced sinus congestion.

4. Hands on the cheeks and nose

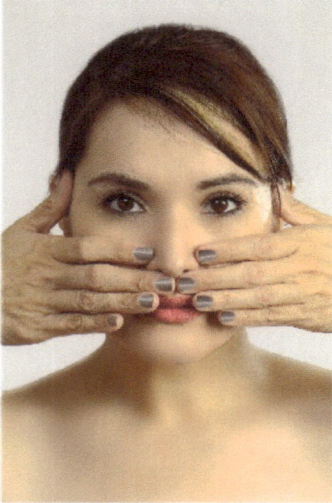

Figure 7 working on self

Place your hands under the eyes. Gentle touch both sides of the mouth. **Allow the energy to flow through your body. Imagine it. Feel it. And make it real. Hold the position and run energy for 5 minutes.** Again, a difficult position to hold on one's own face. I recommend doing it while lying down on a bed or a wide massage table so you can rest your elbows on pillows placed beside your head and shoulders. If you are not able to reach the correct position, do not worry. Place your hands so you are comfortable and set your intention for your fingers to touch the sides of your mouth and lips. Imagine you can reach, touch and be comfortable. Hold the position and run energy for 5 minutes. The position rejuvenates the skin of the cheeks. It increases lip fullness. It removes wrinkles on and above the upper lip.

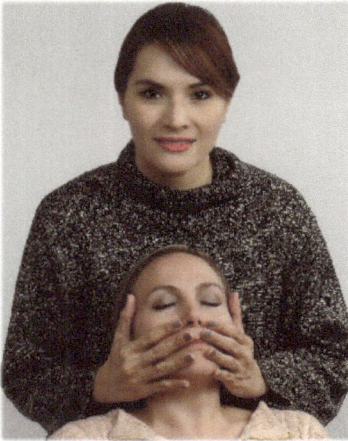

Figure 8 working on client

While working on a client the position is quite easy to hold.

Positive outcomes

The position covers several lymph nodes. Hence it boosts the Lymphatic System. As well, it may ease sinus congestion. It may reduce toothaches. And it may reduce hearing loss.

5. Hands on the chin and the top of the head

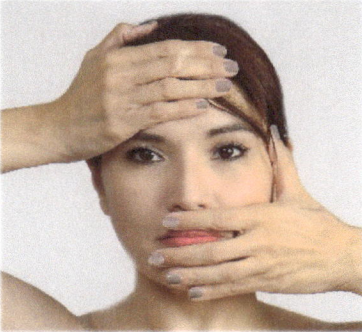

Figure 9 working on self

For this position, find a comfortable place to lie down and use a couple of pillows for support. Cup the chin, place one finger under the nose. Place the index finger on the upper lip, the middle finger on the chin, the ring finger, and pinky under the chin. The thumb rests near the corner of the eye. One hand covers the bottom of the face. The other hand covers the forehead. Cover as much of the face as you can. Allow the energy to flow through your body. Imagine it. Feel it. And make it real. Hold the position and run energy for 5 minutes.

45

The position reinforces most of the previous positions. It boosts the lymph nodes on the chin and relaxes the entire face. It energizes the sub-layers of the skin, removing worn collagen and allowing new collagen to grow.

6. Mirror of the previous hand position

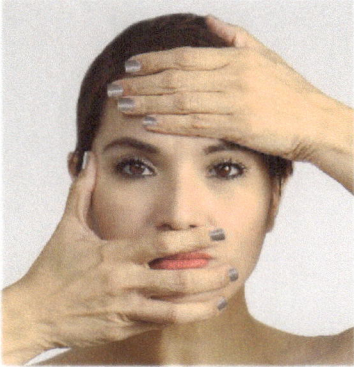

Figure 10 working on self

The sequence of these two positions is really powerful. They reinforce all the previous positions, leading the energy to go to work at a deep level.

Remember, you are doing energy work. Do you feel the energy? Are your hands warm? Are they relaxed? Are you focusing on the lymphatic system? Do you feel the energy flow going through your body? Are you focused on the intention to have beautiful skin, healthy skin, and smooth skin? Experience! Wonder! Enjoy!

7. Hands between the breasts

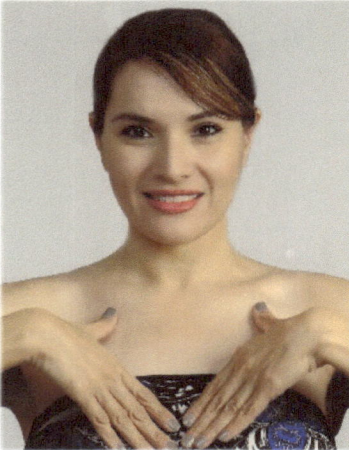

Figure 11 working on self

Place your thumbs on your collar bones and your fingertips on the top of the sternum and move upward, ever so lightly. The position covers the lymph nodes above and below the collar bone. The fingers rest on the thorax, pointing to the thymus gland.

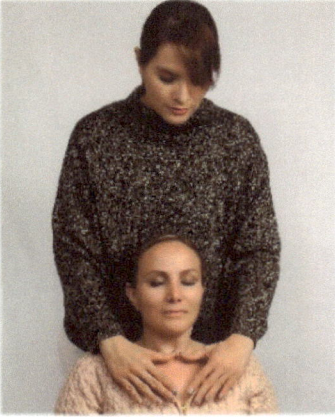

Figure 12 working on client

The position reduces and
removes wrinkles that start in the neck and on the chest. It smoothens crinkled and crepey skin on the chest above the breasts. Allow and feel the energy flow through your whole body. Imagine it. Feel it. And make it real. Hold the position and run energy for 5 minutes.

Positive outcomes

Running energy while focusing on the hand position shown here boosts the lymphatic system. The thymus gland plays a significant role in your overall long-term health.

8. Hands under the armpits

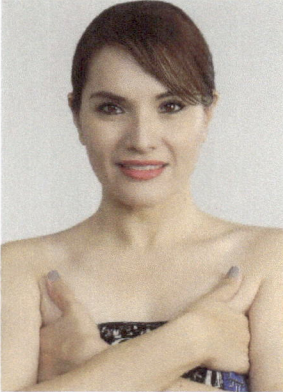

Figure 13 working on self

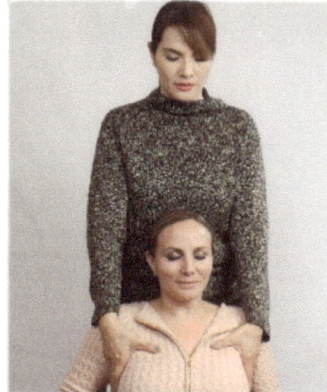

Figure 14 working on client

Place your hands under your armpits with the palms of your hands towards the breasts. Your hands are in contact with the lymph nodes under the arm and on the outside of the breast area. Avoid cupping the breasts. The position boosts the lymphatic system. Allow the energy to flow through your body. Imagine it. Feel it. And make it real. Hold the position and run energy for 5 minutes.

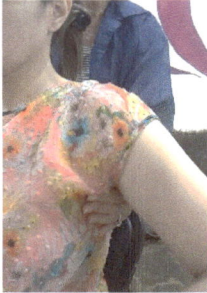

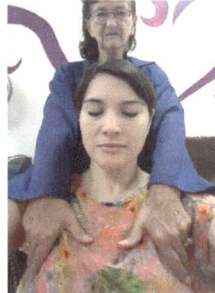

While working with a client there are two ways to do the 'hands under the armpits' position as shown in these pictures. When using the position on the left, stand behind the client who is sitting down. Place open hands from behind the client under the armpit, gently lift and pull. When using the position on the right, the client may be in a sitting or reclining position. In this case, the palms of the hands are toward the client's chest. To start with, practice with someone you know well to find a level of comfort for both of you.

9. Hands on the neck and chest

Place your thumbs on the side of the neck. Rest your index fingers on the collar bone and the tips of your fingers on the breastbone. Place your thumb behind the neck and keep your fingers in front. Your hands are now in contact with the lymph nodes above and below the collar bone. Now gently lift, pulling upwards. The position reduces and removes wrinkles from the chest and neck. Allow the energy to flow through your body. Imagine it. Feel it. And make it real. Hold the position and run energy for 5 minutes. The 'hands on neck and chest' position are much easier to hold when working on a client.

Now you will feel very relaxed. You feel rejuvenated and happy. Your face is glowing and your wrinkles have been greatly reduced. Over the next 3 to 6 days you may notice they will reduce even more.

Towards the end of the last position, you will make a client more comfortable when you tell her the session is almost complete. When you are finished invite her to stay in a relaxed position for a while and get up whenever she feels ready to go.

Basically what we are doing is energy healing on your face and chest for an hour. We like to think of it as **Energetic Pampering.**

QFL MEDITATION

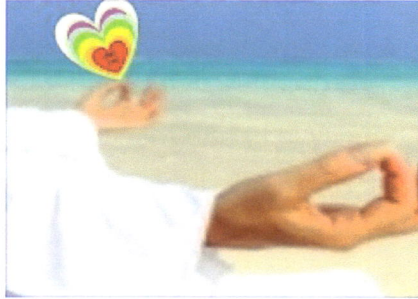

Sit in a comfortable position facing a pleasing picture on your wall.
Imagine you are in one of your favorite places.
Close your eyes and breathe a little more slowly than normal.
Bring your focus behind your eyes.
Place your hands palms upward with thumb and ring finger touching.
Allow your body to relax.
Open your eyes and look at the pleasing picture on the wall in front of you.
Smile.
Close your eyes again and as you do so allow your body to relax even more.
Draw your attention to the skin on your face and your neck.
Feel your smile
Imagine yourself youth-full, relaxed, full of energy and vibrant.
Feel it…. See it… and make it real.

Every cell in your skin is smiling. Feel that smile.
Breathe in the energy, and breathe out youthfulness
through every pore of your skin.
Do this for 2 more minutes.

Now when you are ready, slowly open your eyes and look
again at the pleasant picture on the wall in front of you.

Smile.

AUTHOR'S NOTE

Doing a Quantum Face-Lift does not guarantee total removal of all wrinkles and scars; it aims to lessen and soften them. Quantum Face-Lift is energy work, using a light touch or a near touch. If working with a client, always ask the client's permission to touch sensitive areas of the face, underarms, and chest.

ABOUT THE AUTHOR

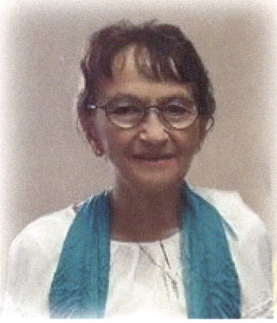

Trudy is an Energy Healing practitioner and instructor. Hands-on healing was part of her childhood experience. She imitated her mother's healing techniques. When her pet dog and other animals were ill with minor issues, she helped to heal them. In her extended family, there were aunts and uncles who also were skilled healers. Today she practices healing modalities including Quantum Touch, Reiki, Psych-K, The Emotion Codes, and Dowsing.

Trudy is a dynamic leader. She engages her audience to participate and enhance their learning experience. We invite you to attend a workshop and you will personally experience the positive outcomes of energy healing: rejuvenation, and anti-aging. It will also provide an opportunity to learn self-healing and healing others. She and her husband Everett live in Newmarket, Ontario during the summer months and in Costa Rica in the winter.

About IEHealers: Trudy and Everett

Our healing journey began at the Oak & River Retreat at 170 Elmpine Trail, King City, Ontario. We have moved on yet the energy of the oak and the river go wherever we go. Our primary focus is wellness orientation, with an emphasis on active personal participation. We are the facilitators but you do the healing. We are rooted in the age-old wisdom of Hippocrates: "The natural healing force within each one of us is the greatest force in getting well".

The name of our first Retreat was with reference to a 300-year-old oak tree that overlooks the property and the river that flows through it. The Oak and the River each on their own and in combination emit energy that transcends time and space.

The Oak embodies strength and empowerment. The flow of the river and the sound of the water rippling over the rocks reverberates fluidity and flexibility, allowing for a free flow of energetic potential.

There remains a place deep within our hearts where we can go, relax, and soak up the peace, the quiet and the power.

No Limits

Most people experience some partial relief as a result of the techniques we practice. However, the healing process is highly individualistic and results vary a great deal from person to person, even for treatment of the same conditions. To quote Alain Herriott:

"I don't know if this [referring to a medical condition] is possible to heal, but I am willing to see what will happen."

Not for Profit

Our business structure is a not-for-profit sole proprietorship. The facilitators are remunerated according to the Health Industry norm.

We offer an affordable and competitive sliding fee schedule. At the end of each fiscal year, any surplus money is deposited into a Trust Fund, which is used to subsidize those for whom the fee structure is not economically feasible.

DISCLAIMER

In all the work we do, Healing Circles, Workshops, Treatments, Retreats, Distant Healing, we do our utmost to use the healing techniques to the best of our abilities. We offer no guarantees. We can only assure you that we do our best to share what we have to offer. The rest is up to you. Although each of the healing modalities we use is highly effective in promoting maximum health and healing through alternative holistic means, it may not be sufficient intervention for some health-related issues or concerns. The sessions may accelerate healing. If you are on medication, we recommend you work closely with your physician to monitor your need for medications, with the intent to reduce your dependency on them. The information on our website our e-mails, and by phone is not given or intended to be a substitute or replacement for qualified medical advice, diagnosis, or treatment. We are not engaged in rendering professional or medical advice.

Please take responsibility for your own health!

www.ingramcontent.com/pod-product-compliance
Lightning Source LLC
Chambersburg PA
CBHW041227270326
41934CB00004B/186